YOUR KNOWLEDGE HAS VALUE

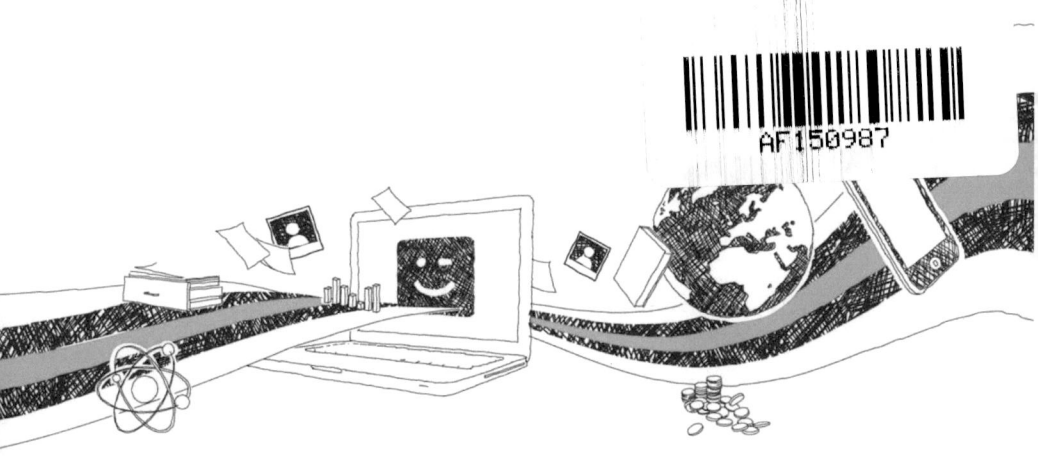

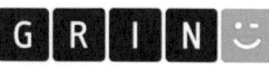

Thembisani Maphosa

Emergency Response to Malnutrition among Returnees,
IDPs and Vulnerable Host Communities in Warrap State,
South Sudan by World Vision

GRIN Publishing

Bibliographic information published by the German National Library:

The German National Library lists this publication in the National Bibliography; detailed bibliographic data are available on the Internet at http://dnb.dnb.de .

Imprint:

Copyright © 2013 GRIN Verlag GmbH
Print and binding: Books on Demand GmbH, Norderstedt Germany
ISBN: 978-3-656-46074-9

This book at GRIN:

http://www.grin.com/en/e-book/230058/emergency-response-to-malnutrition-among-returnees-idps-and-vulnerable

GRIN - Your knowledge has value

Since its foundation in 1998, GRIN has specialized in publishing academic texts by students, college teachers and other academics as e-book and printed book. The website www.grin.com is an ideal platform for presenting term papers, final papers, scientific essays, dissertations and specialist books.

Visit us on the internet:

http://www.grin.com/

http://www.facebook.com/grincom

http://www.twitter.com/grin_com

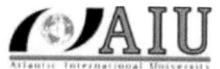

Atlantic International University
A New Age for Distance Learning

THEMBISANI MAPHOSA

COURSE NAME: PROFESSIONAL PROJECT

Emergency Response to Malnutrition among Returnees, IDPs and Vulnerable Host
Communities in Warrap State, South Sudan by World Vision

ATLANTIC INTERNATIONAL UNIVERSITY

Atlantic International University
A New Age for Distance Learning

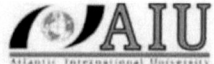

Table of Contents

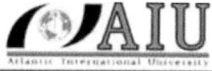
Introduction

South Sudan humanitarian context remains volatile as conflicts and population movement continue amidst worsening food insecurity, and flooding experienced from June to October 2012. In 2012, more than half the population (4.7 million people) were at risk of food insecurity, with over one million people at risk of severe food insecurity, and 3.7 million facing moderate food insecurity. In 2013, 4.6 million South Sudanese are projected to face food insecurity, with 2.3 million South Sudanese likely requiring food assistance according to UN OCHA. This is due to insecurity/conflict, natural disasters, weak commodity markets and insufficient food availability at national level as projected in the annual cereal deficit owing to poor agricultural productivity.

While overall, the numbers of people requiring food assistance figures denote a minor improvement in the country's food security situation compared to 2011/2012; Warrap State is one among 5 states where food insecurity worsened. According to WFP, Warrap has highest rate of severely food insecure households in the country at 66%, with an additional 26% considered moderately food insecure. Access and availability to food remain critical issues. According to a report on food security issued by WFP in August 2012, Warrap currently faces a cereal deficit of almost 60,000 metric tons decreasing food availability for the year ahead. According to FEWSNET, food security in Warrap State is anticipated to remain stressed through to March 2013, after which food security outcomes are anticipated to deteriorate, marking an early start to the lean season.

The most frequent coping mechanisms used by food insecure households includes reducing meal serving size, consumption of cheaper, less preferred food, reducing the number of meals, and limiting adults' consumption. This is evidenced by food consumption rates in Warrap: 30.4% of households have a poor food consumption score meaning that households have low dietary frequency and diversity. About 24% of households in Warrap were considered borderline. The majority (75%) of the severely food insecure group consume less than 4 food groups. Female-headed households are significantly more likely to adopt coping strategies and more severe ones than male-headed ones. While 73% of households with female heads used some coping strategy, 10% less households with male heads reported any strategy.

Inadequate food intake constitutes a major contributing factor to malnutrition. According to WFP, 63% of households in Warrap are considered food deprived, consuming 1301 calories per day, much fewer than FAO's minimum recommended intake for the country of 1717 kcal per person per day to live an active and healthy life. Apart from food availability, cultural dietary taboos and preferences are found to be determinant in influencing nutritional status of children among communities in South

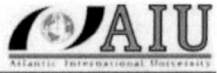
Sudan and have contributed to some of the worst GAM rates since 2010. Women and girls tend to eat last, enjoying the least diet diversity. Young children need at least four meals per day as they are not able to absorb larger quantities in fewer meals. According to a food security survey conducted in 2010, only 4% of under-five children in South Sudan had four or more meals in the previous day, only one third of children consume an adequate diet with the highest proportion in October after the harvest and lowest in February at the beginning of the lean period .

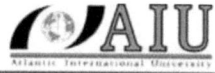
Description

The paper covers a nutrition project implemented by World Vision in Warrap state of South Sudan in the management of malnutrition and food insecurity. It outlines the general components of the community based management of acute malnutrition (CMAM) program in detail i.e. OTP, SC, SFP and community mobilization. It further covers the principal objectives of the project and the activities being carried out to meet those objectives. Capacity building of health staff, routine monitoring and supervision visits are some of the many activities carried out to meet project requirements.

The paper covers a section on WHO Sphere standards and how the project compares to these expected standards and attempts to give variance explanations.

The project has taken great strides in trying to improve the lives of the community and thus this paper documents the progress made to date and makes recommendations accordingly for future reference.

The month of April marked the start of the hunger gap and as part of the project requirements, a SMART nutrition survey was conducted and this is discussed briefly on the paper.

South Sudan is a very young and developing nation so the paper seeks to make recommendations on good health policies and strategies to ensure the nation remains in sync with other nations in providing proper health care practices.

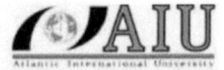
General Analysis

Program Components

According to Valid International the CMAM model has four key components:

- ❖ Community mobilization stimulating the understanding, engagement and participation of the target population.
- ❖ Supplementary feeding programs providing dry take-home rations and routine basic treatment for children with moderate acute malnutrition without complications.
- ❖ Outpatient therapeutic programs providing RUTF and routine treatment using simple medical protocols for children with severe acute malnutrition without complications.
- ❖ Stabilization centers providing inpatient care for acutely malnourished children with medical complications.

The Sphere Project

The Sphere Project was initiated in 1997 by a group of NGOs and the Red Cross and Red Crescent Movement to develop a set of universal minimum standards in core areas of humanitarian response: the Sphere Handbook. The aim of the Handbook is to improve the quality of humanitarian response in situations of disaster and conflict, and to enhance the accountability of the humanitarian system to disaster-affected people.

Table 1: Indicators for Monitoring Feeding Programs

Type of Feeding Program	Indicators	Acceptable (%)	Alarming (%)
Supplementary	Recovery rate	>70	<50
	Death rate	<3	>10
	Defaulting rate	<15	>30
Therapeutic	Recovery rate	>75	<50
	Death rate	<10	>15
	Defaulter rate	<15	>25
	Weight gain (g/kg/day)	>-8	<-8
	Coverage	>50–70	<40
	Mean length of stay	<3–4 weeks	>6 weeks

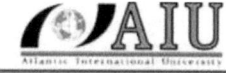
Actualization

Project Title: Emergency Response to Malnutrition among Returnees, IDPs and Vulnerable Host Communities in South Sudan

Principal Objective: To reduce global malnutrition rates among children under five to below 15% in Gogrial East and West, Tonj East and Tonj South and below 10% in Tonj North Counties of Warrap State through immediate response and improved services for prevention of malnutrition

Main Activities:

- Provide services for the treatment of acute malnutrition in children under 5 years, and pregnant and lactating women, people living with HIV, tuberculosis, kala azar and other chronic illnesses
- Provide services for prevention of under-nutrition in children under 5 years, and pregnant and lactating women
- Strengthen nutrition emergency preparedness and response capacity
- Strengthen position of nutrition through advocacy
- Increase the capacity of county health department and WV staff in the management of nutrition interventions

Update on OTP performance indicators Nov 2012 – May 2013

Total number of OTP exits is 1289(out of 1813 Admissions)

Indicator	Sphere standard (%)	Actual performance (%)	Comments
Cure rate	>75	85	Very few cases were referred to the stabilisation centre
Death rate	<10	0	The absolute number of deaths was 2, both recorded in Tonj East
Defaulter rate	<15	14	Most of the defaulters were recorded in Tonj South

The OTP was complemented with the required routine medicines including antibiotic (amoxicillin), antihelmith (Mebendazole/Albendazole), anti-malarial and Vitamin A.

The admissions and discharges are illustrated in the graphs below:

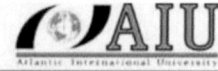
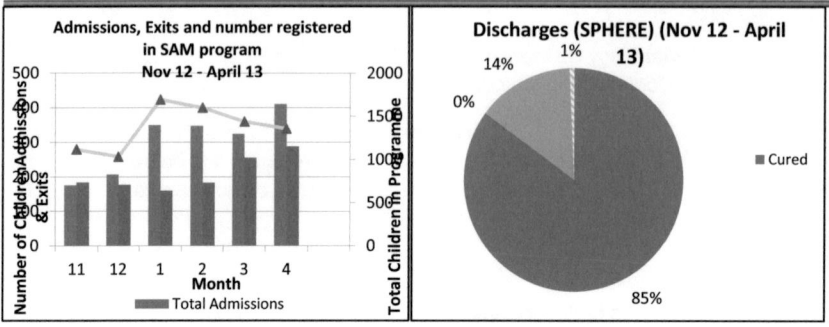

Recovery Rates

The project attained a recovery rate of 85% in the period November 2012 to April 2013. The rate falls within the expected sphere standard (>75%). Majority of the children were managed at the OTP while few cases were referred to SC. Children discharged from OTP were referred to SFP for further management.

Defaulter Rate

The defaulter rate (14%) falls within the expected sphere standard. However the defaulters were followed up in order to determine the reasons for defaulting and mainly to encourage the caregivers to return children and keep them in the programme until full recovery. Majority of the defaulters were recorded in Tonj South and Tonj East.

Mortality Rate

The death rate was within the expected standard sphere target (<10%). The project recorded two deaths during the reporting period. Both deaths occurred in Tonj East and were attributed to late presentation.

Supplementary Feeding Program (SFP)

SFP, which supports children with moderate acute malnutrition without complications, and those discharged from therapeutic treatment, enrolled a total of 6122 children under five years of age. Majority of the children were expected to be admitted to the blanket supplementary feeding program (BSFP) from April (*beginning of the hunger gap*) however enrolment was postponed to May because the fortified supplementary food had not been received from World Food Program (WFP). The supplement food is provided through the Food Aid programme.

All counties were currently screening children for both severe and moderate acute malnutrition. Children with moderate acute malnutrition will receive food packages under

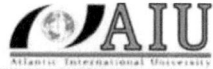
the targeted supplementary feeding program (TSFP) while children below 36 months will be managed under BSFP.

Community Mobilization

Community outreach volunteers were identified and trained in various aspects of the project in an effort to build their capacity in conducting mobilization and active case finding. The community volunteers continuously screened children within the community as evidenced by admissions to both SFP and OTP programmes. The community outreach volunteers also conducted nutrition and health education within the community while the nutrition monitors and the community health workers conducted the education during distributions at OTP/SFP points. All beneficiaries to the various programme components received health and nutrition education.

SMART Survey

SMART nutrition surveys were conducted to measure the impact of the hunger gap on the community. The data collection tool was divided into the following five sections:

i.   Anthropometric questionnaire
ii. Mortality questionnaire
iii. Infant and young child feeding questionnaire
iv. Water and sanitation questionnaire
v.   Food security and livelihoods questionnaire

The survey reports are under compilation, however preliminary results indicated an increased prevalence of global acute malnutrition compared to the same period last year. The prevalence in almost all the counties was above the acceptable threshold according to WHO standards.

Project summary in pictures

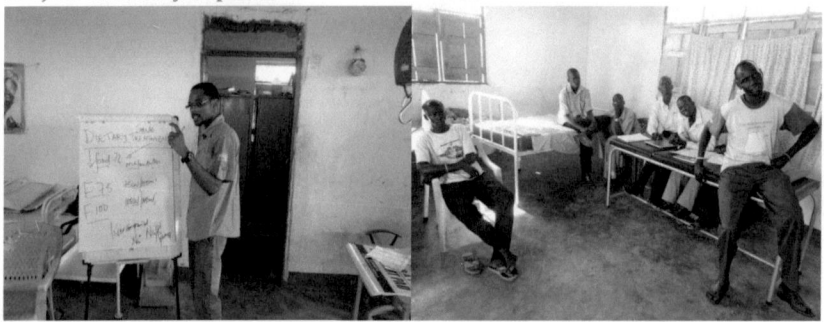

Capacity building of health staff in Tonj North

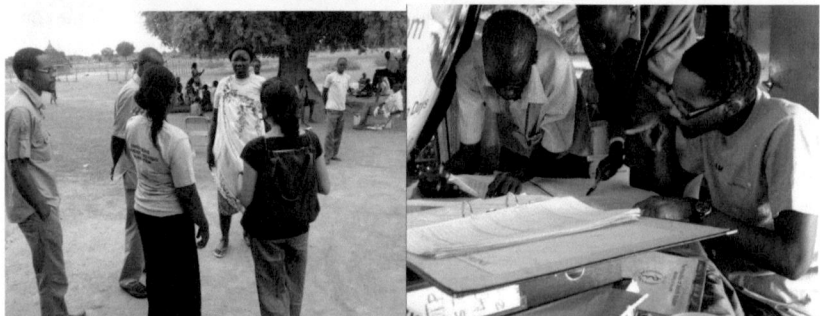

Project monitoring and evaluation in Paraksika PHCC (left) and Pagol PHCC (right) Tonj North

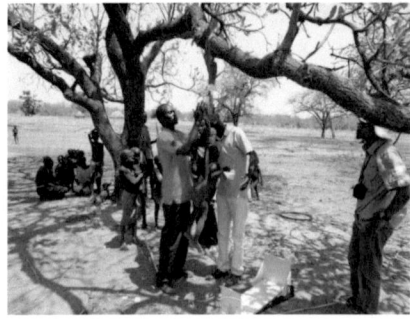 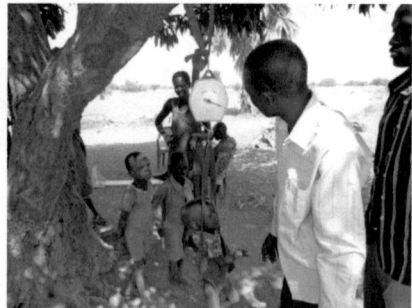

SMART Nutrition Survey in Tonj North (left) & Gogrial East (right)

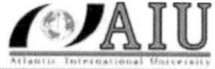
Discussion

As discussed in the previous section, defaulter rate is below the sphere standards but with reference to other indicators it is generally high. The program is faced with this challenge owing to the long distances that beneficiaries have to travel to get to the OTP sites. People have to walk long distances in the scotching sun to get to the health facilities. Most of the primary health care centers (PHCCs) in the area were constructed by World Vision and still these are not enough to sustain everyone, hence there is need for the government to construct more permanent health service delivery structures.

The international humanitarian agencies are doing a very good job in helping communities in South Sudan, but this has negative impact on most communities and to some extent the leadership. People are now so dependent on aid that they can hardly think 'outside the box'. There is a vast amount of idle land that can be used for agriculture yet people still face challenges of food insecurity and malnutrition. Others are even convinced that it's their right to be given food by WFP.

Literacy levels are very low among most communities hence this makes it difficult even to apply the behavior change communication strategy. Most people don't really find it necessary to change their traditional practices. They believe that foreigners are colonizing them and infiltrating them with their alien cultures. Water has been made readily available to most communities through drilling of boreholes but hand washing still remains an uncommon practice to many.

Millennium Development Goals (MDGs)

According to Waage, Jeff, et al, (2010) progress towards reaching the goals has been uneven. Some countries have achieved many of the goals, while others are not on track to realize any. A UN conference in September 2010 reviewed progress to date and concluded with the adoption of a global action plan to achieve the eight anti-poverty goals by their 2015 target date. Achieving these benchmarks hinges on sound and effective health policies. However having these policies alone will not bring change, and there is need for government and stakeholder commitment. There were also new commitments on women's and children's health, and new initiatives in the worldwide battle against poverty, hunger, and disease. The year 2015 is fast approaching thus making it highly unlikely that most of the goals will be achieved. A number of factors have contributed greatly towards slowing progress with the global economic crisis and climate change being the 'chief culprits'.

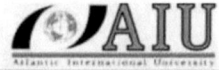
According to UNDP (www.sd.undp.org/mdg_fact.htm) recent surveys have shed light on the massive level of poverty and deplorable human development situation in South Sudan. The country endured years of armed conflict which only ended in 2005, five years after the adoption of the Millennium Declaration. The start of work towards these goals was therefore delayed and started from a very low baseline: realistically, most will not be met by 2015 unless an accelerated effort is made to address the challenges posed by the current state of conflict and fragility in South Sudan. National capacities and institutions need to be strengthened to manage initiatives oriented to achieving the MDGs.

The government is believed to have an estimated seven years of oil revenue left with which it can fund some of the major investments necessary in social services, infrastructure and agriculture. UNDP is providing technical advice to planning processes, building institutional capacity, and helping to support the development of inclusive economic growth strategies that promote employment, livelihoods and effective delivery of services and reduce inequalities and marginalization of the poor and vulnerable groups.

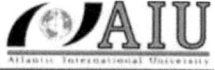
General Recommendations

- ❖ There is a need to focus on the marginalised group (women and girls) in developmental projects. Donor countries should invest in projects that increase girl's completion of secondary school and compete with their male counterparts in the job industry.
- ❖ Strengthen the existing OTPs and SCs in terms of effective community outreach and logistics this can be achieved through increasing the number of SCs and OTPs in the existing CMAM counties and payams considering population density and accessibility.
- ❖ Establish government of South Sudan (GoSS) commitment for increasing its share of funding, some of the income realized from oil export can be used to complement the health budget.
- ❖ Work closely with agriculture and food security sectors to improve production of locally available weaning foods
- ❖ Support and strengthen civil society organizations and community based organizations.
- ❖ Enforce a law that every child in the school going age be at school.
- ❖ The government should invest in large scale farming schemes and provide farmers with latest state of the art machinery.
- ❖ Nutrition interventions should be given longer term/ multiyear budgets so as to make an impact rather than the 6-9 months project periods.
- ❖ Develop the needed national human resource capacity and ensure that all personnel in high and influential positions in the ministry have a very strong health background.
- ❖ There is an urgent need to improve environmental sustainability since most communities use firewood as their source of fuel and this degrades the arable land thus affecting agricultural productivity.
- ❖ Improve personal hygiene among communities.
- ❖ Increase male involvement in management of malnutrition and infant and young child feeding related issues.
- ❖ Logistical processes of procuring and distributing RUTF should be improved to avoid stock outs.
- ❖ Home visit follow up should be strengthened; use of mothers groups is fine but not as effective as home visit.
- ❖ Incentives for nutrition monitors should be increased because these cadres assist in strengthening local capacity at community level.
- ❖ Conduct lessons learnt sessions every end of month or quarter.

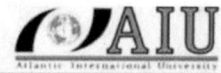
Conclusion

Limited dietary diversity was one of the critical findings of the SMART nutrition survey conducted in April. Majority of the world's poorest communities are rural farmers, however agriculture is not given strong emphasis in the MDGs. South Sudan has a vast portion of fertile land that can easily be exploited for agricultural activities and unless this is done the problem of malnutrition is still far from over. There were a lot of cases of compromised hygiene in most communities visited during the survey and this explains the prevalence of eye infections and diarrhea. Communities should be empowered on good hygiene standards through intensive WASH interventions.

Most of the work in the health and nutrition sector is in the hands of NGOs and private sector and this impact negatively on sustainability of projects due to recurrent staff turnovers as these employees are working on contractual basis. The government has a mandate of empowering the local staff in the field of health and nutrition in order to have continuity and scale up operations. One way of doing this will be providing outstanding students with comprehensive scholarships to further their education in universities outside the country.

The referral pathway of severe complicated cases to the stabilization center is usually a bottleneck as a result of the bad transport network as most of the communities are poor and don't afford to hike to the stabilization centers. Project quality is compromised with these challenges and this can only be improved by moving the resources closer to the masses.

Although the country, just like many others looks set to miss the 2015 MDG deadline, there is still great potential beyond this date owing to the country's well-articulated health strategic plan (2011-2015).

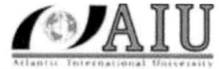

References

1. American Journal of Epidemiology 2001 by the Johns Hopkins University Bloomberg School of Public Health Vol. 154, No. 12 USA

2. FEWSNET, South Sudan Food Security Outlook July to December 2012 http://www.fews.net/docs/Publications/South_Sudan_OL_2012_07_final.pdf

3. UNICEF Fact Sheet: http://www.unicef.org/sudan/UNICEF_Sudan_health_and_nutrition_fact_sheet

4. Valid International. 2006. *Community-based Therapeutic Care. A Field Manual.* 1st edition. Oxford, UK: Valid International. http://www.fantaproject.org/ctc/manual2006.shtml.

5. Waage, Jeff, et al, (18 September 2010). "The Millennium Development Goals: a cross-sectoral analysis and principles for goal setting after 2015

6. World Health Organization (2012) National Health accounts retrieved from: http://www.who.int/nha/use/en/

7. WHO/FAO release independent Expert Report on diet and chronic disease". World Health Organization. Retrieved 21 February 2011.

8. WHO/WFP/SCN/UNICEF Joint Statement on CMAM, 2007.

9. www.thelancet.com/journals/lancet/article/PIIS0140-6736(10)61196-8/fulltext

10. www.sd.undp.org/mdg_fact.htm

11. www.unocha.org/south-sudan